The Magic of Grapes

To Cure and Heal

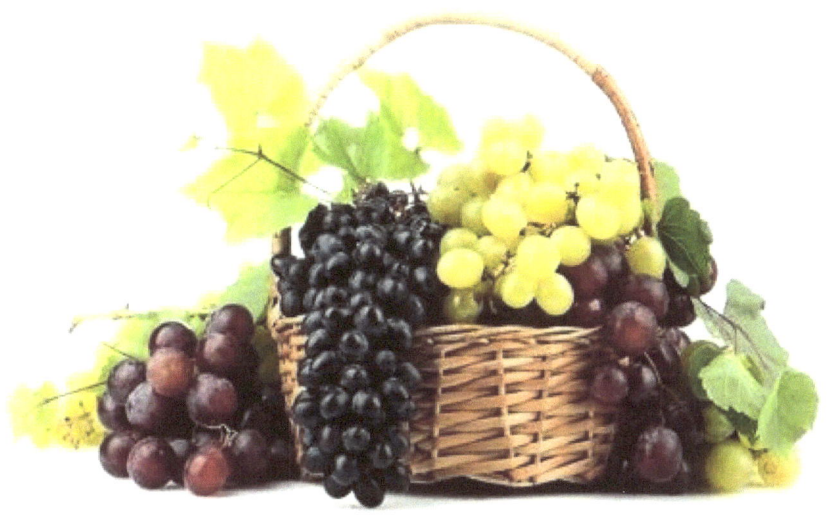

Dueep Jyot Singh

Natural Remedy Series

Mendon Cottage Books

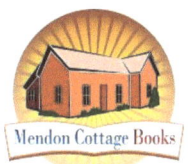

JD-Biz Publishing

Disclaimer

The information is this book is provided for informational purposes only. It is not intended to be used and medical advice or a substitute for proper medical treatment by a qualified health care provider. The information is believed to be accurate as presented based on research by the author.

The contents have not been evaluated by the U.S. Food and Drug Administration or any other Government or Health Organization and the contents in this book are not to be used to treat cure or prevent disease.

The author or publisher is not responsible for the use or safety of any diet, procedure or treatment mentioned in this book. The author or publisher is not responsible for errors or omissions that may exist.

Warning

The Book is for informational purposes only and before taking on any diet, treatment or medical procedure, it is recommended to consult with your primary health care provider.

Our books are available at

1. Amazon.com
2. Barnes and Noble
3. Itunes
4. Kobo
5. Smashwords
6. Google Play Books

Table of Contents

Introduction

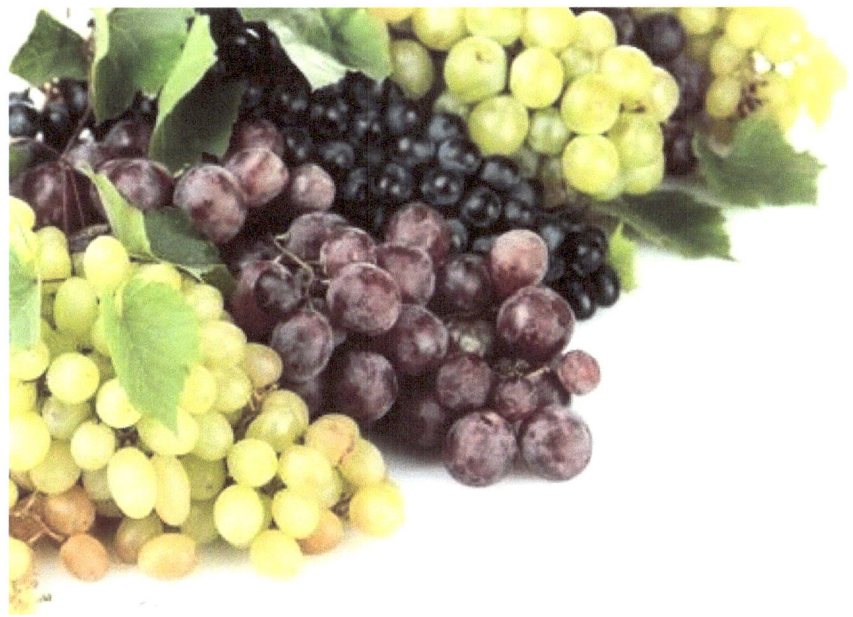

The moment you hear the word "grapes", you visualize a bunch of yellow or black – purple delicious, juicy fruit, which you enjoy plucking off their stalks and popping in your appreciated mouth. Believe it or not, grapes are just about the only fruit, which can be eaten in large quantities, without any sort of harmful side effects.

The magic about grapes is that not only is this considered to be an extremely good way which you can cure yourself, but it is also such a good and delicious, easy to eat fruit, that even fussy and finicky eaters who touch fruits and vegetables very rarely cannot resist a fistful of grapes.

The history of grapes goes back as long as mankind existed. In prehistoric times, grapes were gathered in the jungles, before man decided to cultivate them in his vineyards or gardens.

The Bible says that Noah grew grapes on his farm. But before that, the classical age of Greece had already assigned a God Dionysius, as the God of grapes and wine, and you can see him sporting around with the grape vine leaves around his head as he blesses his worshipers with the gift of the grapes – wine. The Romans called him Bacchus.

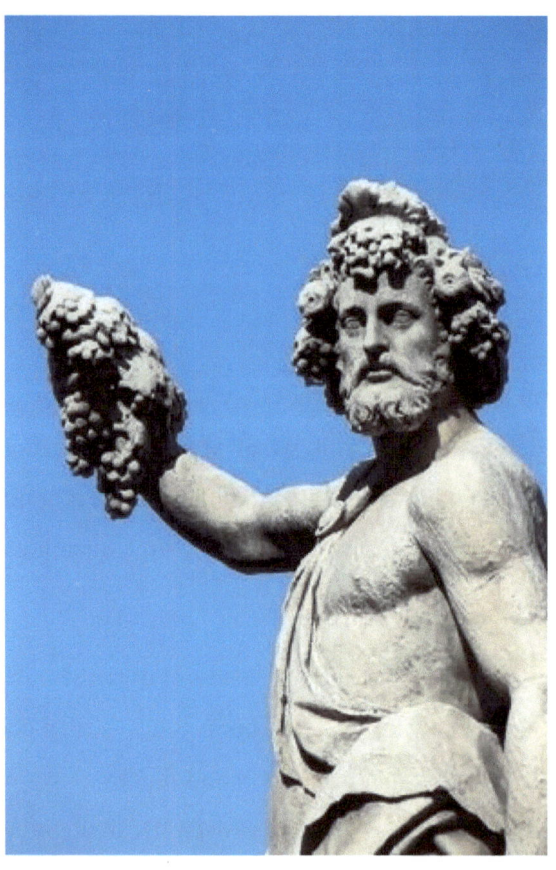

So when did wine get associated with grapes? An old legend talks about a Georgian princess who was suffering from toothache *around 8000 years ago*. No dentist would do anything for her, so being a delicate dainty darling, she said that she was going to kill herself because she could not bear the pain. So she went around looking for something to eat, which would put her out of her misery.

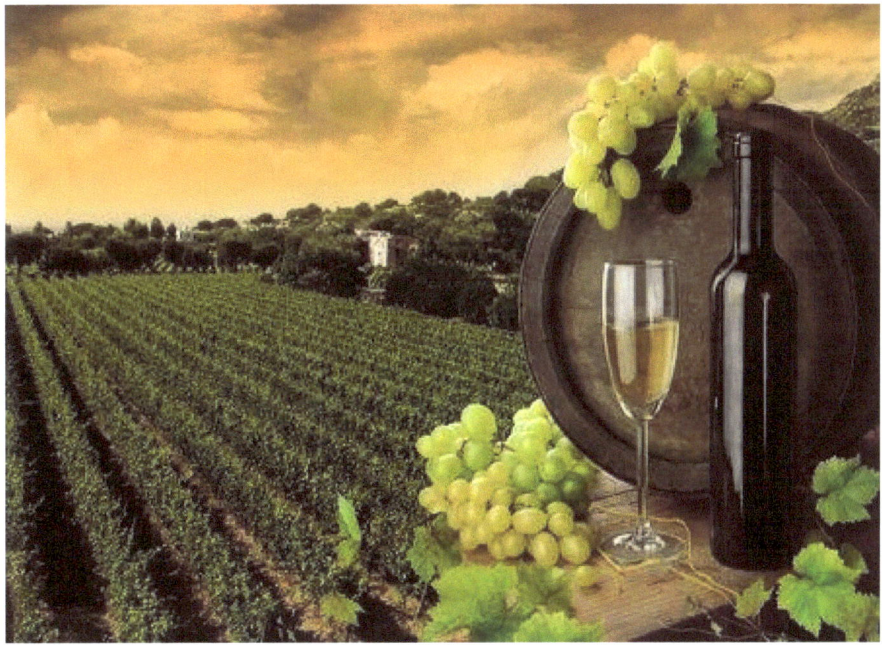

Now one of her could not care less slaves had left some grape juice neglected in an earthenware pot, and it had been fermenting over a long time in its corner. Naturally, it gave out the fermenting aroma of grape wine, which no one in that land had smelled before. So the Princess grabbed this pot, and drank everything and grew tipsy.

I am sure, she woke up with a hangover, but according to her, her toothache was gone and she had slept and dreamt pleasantly of no pain. Well, that was how people began to think about the juice of the grape in its fermented form.

In the same way, poetry, talking about the wine of Shiraz, going back more than 4000 years ago, speaks about the importance of wine in the old Oriental legends.

Wine can be made from almost any vegetable or fruit, yes, I have heard of people making wine from vegetables too, but that is rather an insult to the not so humble grape, because this berry is best suited to give you enough of juice, to make delicious sparkling wine, which can either be champagne, or can be ordinary table wine. Also, wine, if not made from farm grown grapes ripen in the sun in their vineyards, I consider to be sacrilege, and really not worth appreciating, or savoring.

Mark Twain in his hilarious book "Innocents abroad" talks about enjoying the adventure of he and his friends raiding an Italian vineyard at night, when they reach Italy. Now that should have been quite an intoxicating experience.

My father still remembers with nostalgia, eating the local, delicious and juicy grapes of California, which he compares favorably with the grapes of France. Most of all, he enjoys that absolutely Huge bowl full of their locally produced non-hybrid grapes, left in his hotel room, by the compliment of the management even though the wine bottle was not present.

 But he did not miss the wine, [fruit and wine was the norm in European hotels, especially in Italy and in France, where the management also gifted you an assortment of local cheeses, with their compliments] because he had his hands full of the original deal!

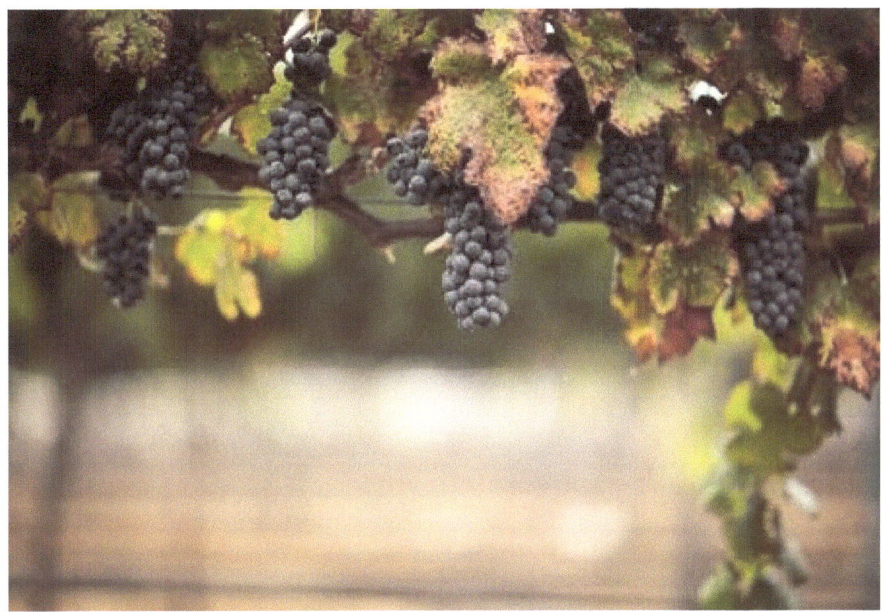

This was in the 60s, so grape hybrids, – which concentrate on weight and volume rather than taste and flavor, which are sacrificed during the hybridizing process – were not so much in vogue in Californian vineyards at that time.

Apart from eating grapes, fresh off the vine, you can also eat them in grape jam and in grape vinegar. Also, raisins and sultanas are made up of seed and seed less grapes.

The Global Scope of Grapes

The most famous grape vineyards in Europe are in France and Italy. In the USA, California, is well-known for its grape production and so is Australia getting to be known for its high quality wine.

The most popular, expensive and most delicious grape in the East is grown in a place named Chaman [literally – garden] since ancient times. This is in Afghanistan. It is not exported, because the local produce is taken up by local traders, who want to keep this grape to themselves.

Here are some reminiscences about the people of that area. Since ancient times, the medicine in this area has had a Greek influence, thanks to Alexander the great's soldiers, deciding to settle here, around 2000 years ago, and raise families. Instead of going back to Greece, they intermarried with the native women of Gandhaar, which was what that area was called since ancient times, going back to the Mahabharata – guess that age to be 7000 years ago – [this name is reflected in the name of that well-known city *Kandahar*].

I bet they brought this great grape and planted it here, in their garden, in Gandhaar. It is still grown with absolutely no artificial pesticide, and natural fertilizers. According to the farmers, organic fertilizers poison the soil and poison the fruit.

Grapes for Health

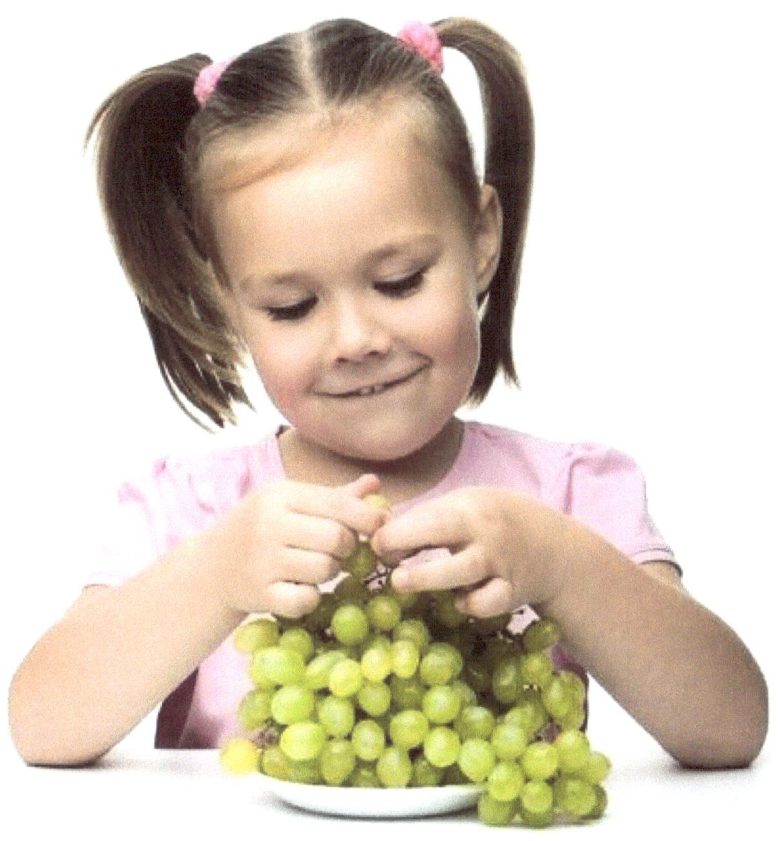

Because of its particular medicinal values, the people of that area using the Greek idea of plenty of sun, good food and no worries, coming down from ancient times used to make sure that any old person, who was getting to be really sick was put into this grape orchard. Along with that he had easy access to other dried fruits, which are grown in abundance in Afghanistan.

He lived in a thatched shed, to shelter him from the sun and the cold in the night. Just one family member replenished his earthen pitcher of water every day, and fed him home baked naan- the local bread – along with bowls full of soup [goat/sheep, chicken meat depending on the financial status of the family, for lunch, as well as for supper.]

This sick old person was then allowed to spend his days in the open air, with healthy food, and eat everything that was growing in the orchards and as much as he could.

The other adults in the family kept their day to day problems and worries and also them away from the ailing member of their family and tribe. That was so that he did not feel any sort of mental responsibility and tension. His care was the responsibility of just one family member, who considered it a matter of pride, when his grandfather came back to the tribe, all hale and hearty.

This was the custom, even up to the 30s and 40s, and I do not know whether this is still being practiced, but the longevity of the people in that area, and their comparative better health is considered to be stuff of legends.

I believe the idea of taking care of a family member came down from ancient Greece traditions, mixed with ancient Indian subcontinent traditions. And then, good food, open air, no medicines, – unless they were herbal remedies, coming down from Greek times and ancient times – cured the ailing aged elder, **98% of the time.**

Naturally grapes played a very important role in his recovery.

Grapes to "Cure" Possible Incurable Diseases

Now let me tell you a real story about the real value of grapes, in helping cure people suffering from cancer. A relative of mine experimented with this cure. She went on to a purely grape diet for three months, while her yes, last stage of cancer was declared incurable by doctors, and told her that she had better go home and live out the rest of her days – which were limited –, eating pain deadening drugs because they were quite sorry and they could not do anything more for her.

So she stopped eating any cereal products, including bread, and started a diet of just grapes and buttermilk.

She survived those three crucial months. In fact, she survived for *18 years* more. But that was because these two items were a part of her diet, along with fresh fruit and vegetables.

Hundred grams of grapes are going to give you 69 kcal of energy, along with carbohydrates, sugars, and plenty of vitamins, including the B complex vitamins, vitamin E, vitamins C, and vitamin K. Along with that, you get elements like magnesium, sodium, potassium, phosphorus, iron, zinc and manganese in grapes. So you can consider this to be a complete health food, to restore all the depleted minerals and vitamins in your body.

Types of Grapes

There are about 140 cultivars of grapes available to us today, coming down from the grapevines of yore. In fact, during war in ancient and medieval times, the farmers used to make sure, that they had some grape plant cuttings, stored away, somewhere, because after the war was over, it would be the job of those cuttings to bring prosperity back to their destroyed farms.

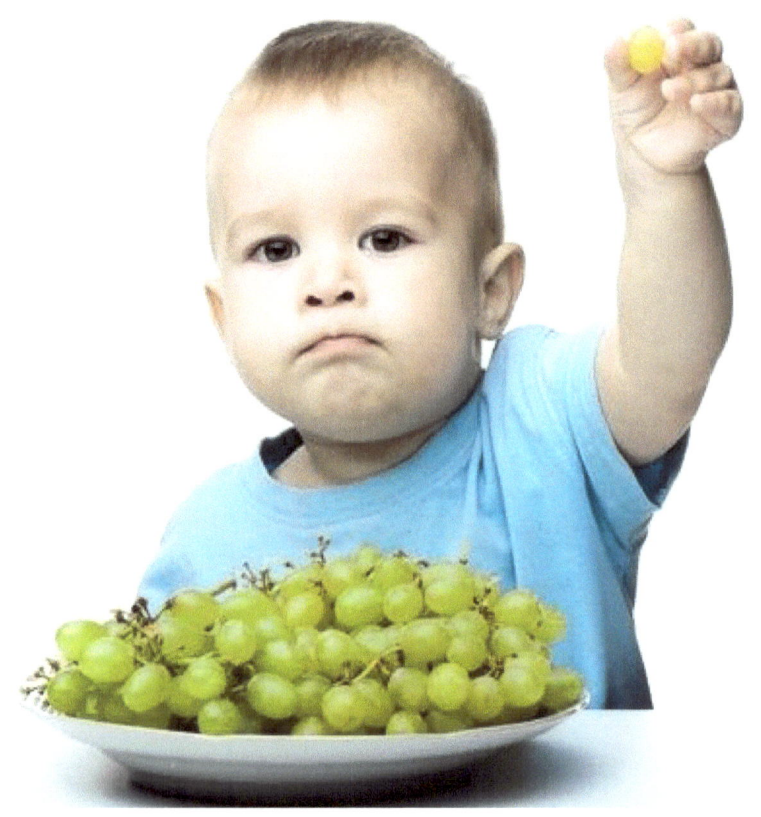

The color of grapes is definitely not restricted to just the ordinary yellow and the Black or Crimson. You have plenty of varieties, giving you pink, green, and even orange grapes. The color of the grape is going to depend on the amount of natural anthocyanins and other actual pigment materials present in them.

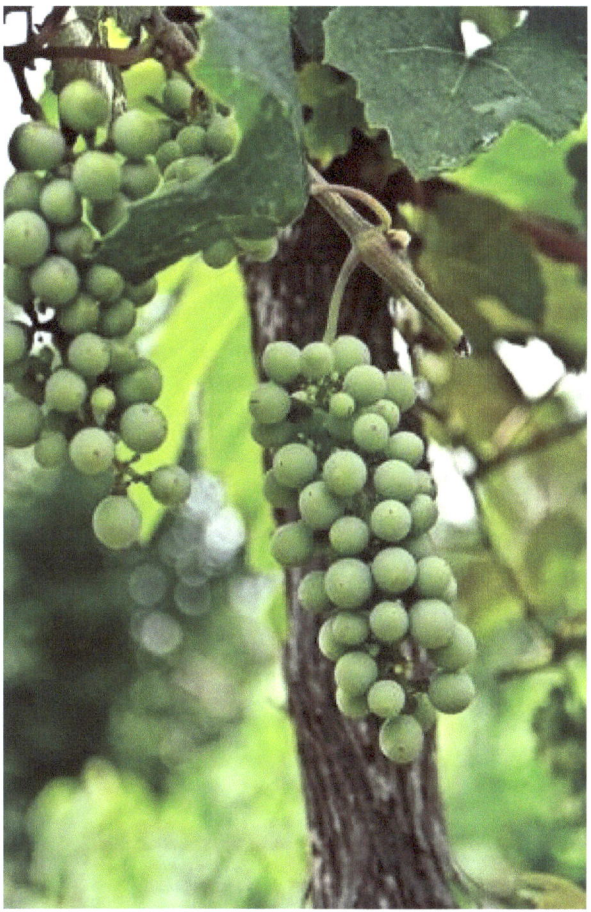

Green Muscadine

Vitis vinifera is the grape extensively grown in Middle East, and in the way. Read your rainy and region. Along with that, the wines produced in Asia and in America comes from Vitis labrusca and the North American native Vitis riparia, which is excellent for jams.

The muscadine grapes are famous for its wine production in France, United States and the Gulf of Mexico. Their scientific name is Vitis rotundifolia. Yes, they are totally rotund and rich in juice.

Vitis amurensis is what the Chaman grapes are. They are grown extensively in Asia, but they came here from Europe – especially from Greece.

Some of the most popular grape varieties, which are planted in France to make their own special wines include Chardonnay, Sauvignon Blank, Grenache, Cabernet Sauvignon, Chardonnay and Riesling.

The ever popular Sultana grape, which is now called the Thompson seedless, as well as the Black Monukka are Vitis vinifera cultivars.

Monukka is the traditional name for dried seedless plants grapes, which can also take the place of raisins in Eastern cuisine and herbal remedies. Many of the ancient herbal medicines and traditions start with – *take four Monukkas and then…*

Aha, says the patient to himself, "I need to go and search for the black dried large variety of grapes which do not have seeds in them. That is what the wise ancient well-versed in herbal lore meant when he told me to eat this remedy with Monukkas."

Spain leads the word today, in grape cultivation. It is followed by France and Italy. However China tops the world in producing grapes, followed by the United States and then Italy. 67,067,128 metric tons of grapes were produced all over the world in 2012.

Difference between Wine Grapes and Table Grapes

Wine grapes are sweeter, because they have a larger sugar content. Table grapes are different cultivars altogether. These grapes ready for the table have seedless grapes, and they are larger in size. Their skin is thinner than wine grapes.

Grapes which are used in making wine are smaller in size, but juicier in content. They also have seeds in them. That is why they are used to make wine, because all the aroma of the wine comes from the skin. So if you find yourself making wine from grapes, which are completely skinned, you are going to wonder where the aroma went!

The table grapes definitely do not have excessive sugar content, but because they are seedless, they are used to make what is now being sold as commercially packaged and produced "grape juice – hundred percent natural product."

Seriously speaking, this hundred percent natural product, is also going to be mixed up with fillers and additives to make up the weight. Also, you are going to find chemical preservatives added to this supposedly hundred percent natural product, in order to increase its shelf life.

Also, people can get away with wines made from table grapes, by saying that they have just made them for private consumption, and thus they do not have to bother about strict and stringent quality testing rules from government officials.

How Do You Grow Grapes?

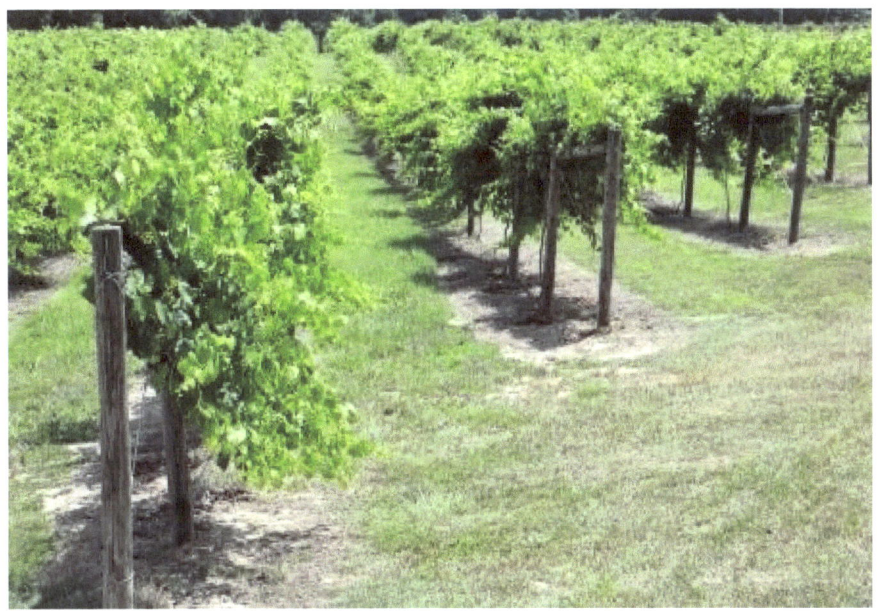

Grapes are now being popularly grown with the help of cultivars, especially with seedless plants cultivars. Grape cuttings are placed in prepared soil, and vegetative propagation is done to grow a seedless plant.

Many people are under the impression that grapes cannot bear extreme temperatures, and especially they do not grow in areas where there is plenty of frost in the winter, but there is not true in the 21st century. We have Venus as well as Reliance Varieties of grapes, which have been grown successfully in areas which are considered to be rather cold, especially South Ontario and the northeastern part of the United States.

Grapes are perennial plants, which grow on vines, with woody stems. Once your grape arbor has decided to take firm root in the ground, you are going to find yourself with a plant which is going to last for the next 40 to 50 years, giving you a rich harvest every year.

Grapes just love the sun that is why you have to make sure that they are planted in an area which is extremely sunny, and is also well moisturized. Also, the soil should be rich in nutrients, and also should be well-drained.

Growing grapes is not something which you do in a day. That is because it is going to take four years for your plants to produce fruits. So make sure that you know that this is a long-term commitment, which is going to help you get the best results for all your hard work.

The growing season is going to depend on the variety of the grapes that you are cultivating. Also, the climate is going to have a major effect on your grapes.

Best Climate for Grapes

Humidity, rainfall, temperature, as well as the amount of sunshine are all important and relevant factors which are going to make all the difference between a good grape crop or a wasted effort for this year. Extreme climates like desert areas, and extremely cold climates are not conducive to good grape growing. The idea is that the grape is going to ripen in plenty of sun.

The grape cuttings need to be planted after the frost is over, so that the chutes can start sprouting. Also, there should be plenty of sun, and plenty of water to allow these plans to grow and flourish. You may want to choose either the early spring, or late spring and the onset of summer to plant your grapes.

Best Soil for Grapes

Like I said before, there should be plenty of nutrients, and organic minerals already present in the soil, which is going to come through organic fertilizer. The soil should be able to retain water, and also, it should also have the ability to allow it to drain away. Any water which is left standing in the soil is going to cause root rot.

Grapes from Seeds or from Young Vines?

I would suggest that you go to the nearest nursery, and asked them for their suggestions or advice for the best time as well as the species which you want to plant in your garden. Bring, young grape vines from the nursery, and plant immediately. If you leave them to dry instead of planting them, you are going to find that your plants are not going to grow.

If you cannot plant them immediately, just make a shallow trench in the soil, and cover the roots of the plant. Then water that soil so that it keeps the soil moist.

Grapes need plenty of area to grow and that is why you need to have a distance of at least 10 feet between your grapevines. That is because the roots are going to spread underground all over the place.

If you want to grow grapes from grape seeds, that is a different proposition altogether, because my gardener said that that was very difficult and he has been trying to do that for the last four years. Maybe people are successful in growing grapes from seeds, if the weather is inclement, and the soil is ready along with the climate and moisture content in the prepared bed.

Plenty of Water

Along with some, grapes need lots of water. So remember to water them regularly, especially during the first six months, when they are going to do most of their growing. Also, remember that the water should be drained properly before you go on to another watering session of your grapes.

Organic manure is of course the best food for your grapes. You may want to make your own compost from farmyard manure or you can just add a shovel full from a compost heap.

The healthiest grapevines are going to have healthy dark green leaves. The soil depth should be 5 to 6 inches. Add another 2 inches of organic material as a fertilizer. Then water the plant. This is going to allow the fertilizer to get absorbed in the soil.

Making a Trellis for Your Vine
Grapevines just need support!

A grape vine is quite a frail and flimsy thing, even though it is the thing of beauty and a joy forever. That is why it needs adequate support. Make sure that your trellises for support are made up of wood or bamboo. You need at least 8 feet of trellis. This release needs to be strong. No metal trellises, please, because the coming of winter, your grapes are going to freeze, thanks to the cold metal and in summer, they are going to boil. Not good.

Prune all the damaged buds after the onset of winter, so that they do not take up all the extra food from the rest of the healthy buds. You may also want to prune the new shoots as they spring up every spring, on the sides of your woody grape stem. You do not want them to prevent the main grape stem from growing properly, and in a healthy manner, do you?

Protecting Your Grapes from Birds

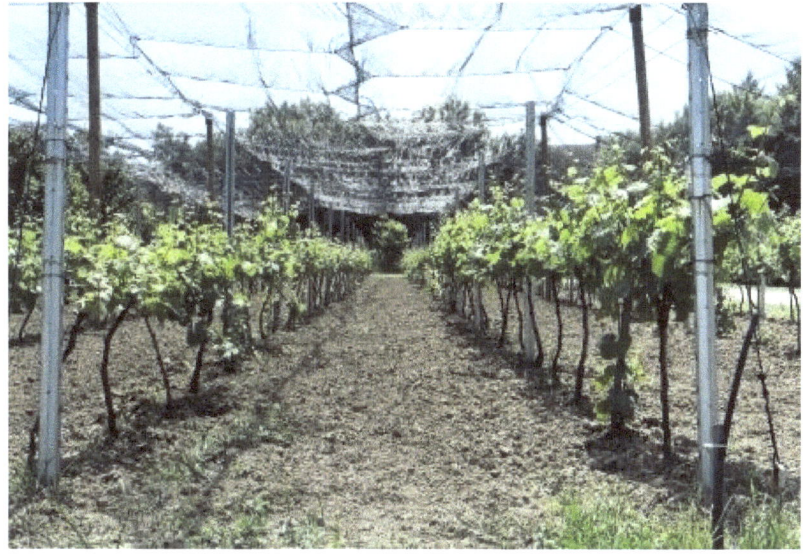

The moment your grapes start ripening, you are going to be subjected to continuous insect and bird attacks. That is why you need to protect your fruit with plastic netting. Fungus infections can be prevented by sprinkling your grape leaves and plant with natural and organic pesticides.

You may want to put up a large bird scarecrow to scare away smaller birds. Or perhaps a plastic dangerous looking snake.

Harvesting Your Grape Yield

This is the most interesting part of growing grapes. The whole community is definitely going to be interested in harvesting the grapes, and eating them. Fresh off the vine, these juicy grapes are definitely the fruit of the gods.

When the lower sections of the grapes show a ripe color, you should get ready to harvest them. So gather the clan together, get some baskets ready and get set go. You just need a small pair of scissors, and your basket on your arm. Just grab the bunch of grapes from their stalks, snip with one hand and put in the basket with the other hand.

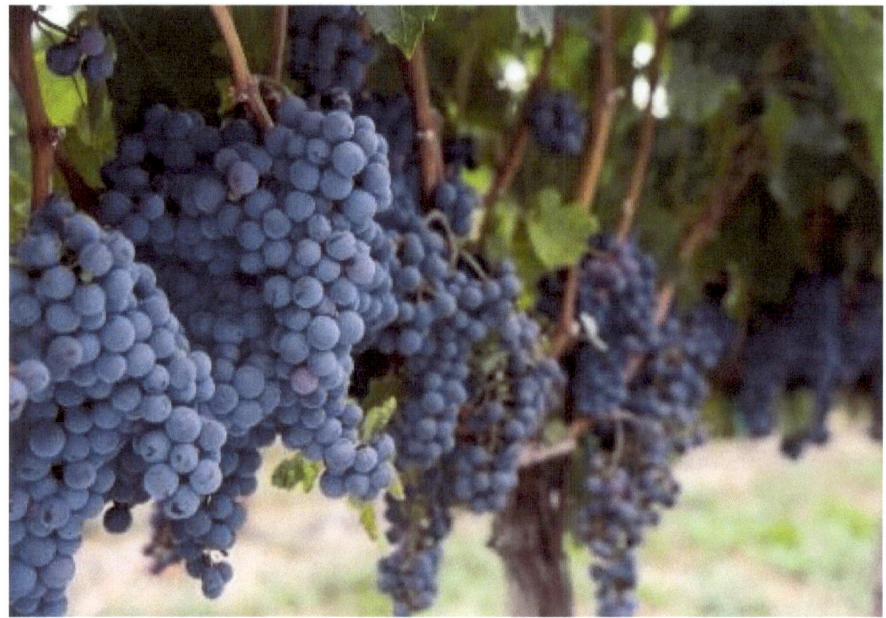

Difference between Sultanas, Raisins, and Grapes

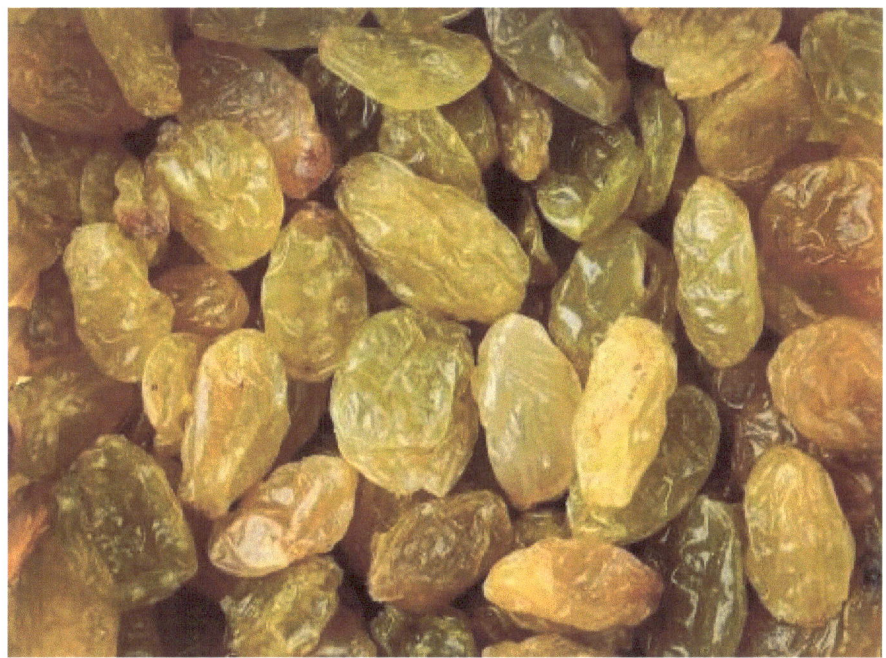

Raisins

The moment you hear about raisins, you think about dried grapes. Grapes are the juicy fruits that you pick off the vine or grab off the market shelves. Any dried grape – also known as "dried vine fruit" in the EU – can be called a raisin in the USA or in the UK. Raisin actually is the French word for a single grape. The bunch is called a grappe , so you request a *grappe de raisins, Oone graap duh rey san*)when you go shopping in France. This word grappe became grape in English.

The sultana is just a dried raisin coming from Turkey, and it is normally bleached in color. Currants, in the UK are dried, Corinth, black grapes, but in the USA, this term is used to describe red currants and black currants, which both happened to be berries, and are definitely not grapes

How to Get Grape Juice?

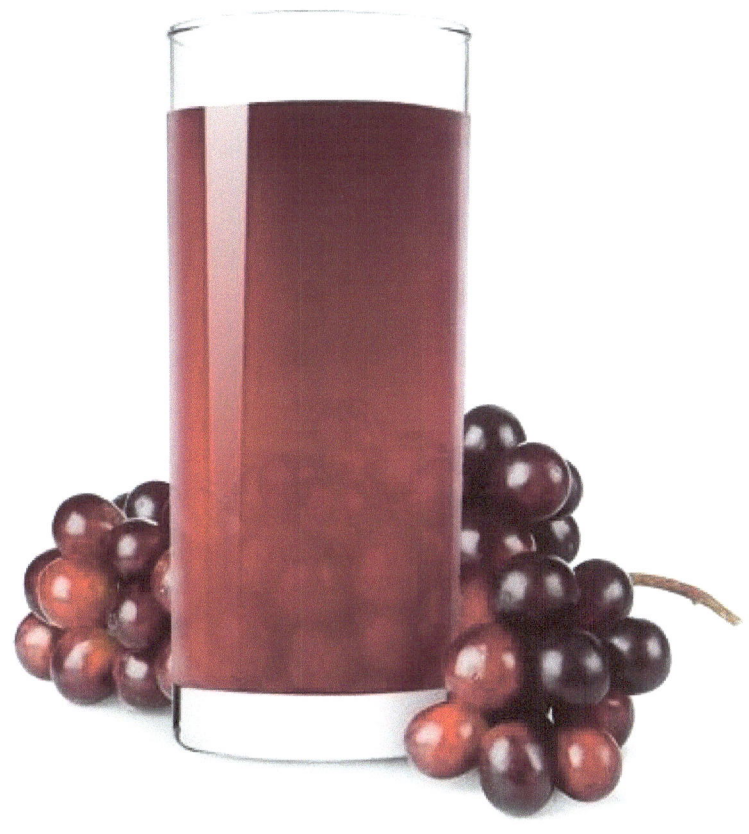

Juice them WITH skin!

Real grape juice is definitely not going to be seeded, and it is going to have the skin in. That is because the seed has plenty of beneficial oil in it. So if you remove the seeds, and the skin, you will just have juice from the pulp.

Winemakers make sure that up to 23% of the grape juice content is made up of seeds, skins, and even stems to make real good quality wine.

The grape juice that you drink in the USA, and which has been packaged commercially is made up of the locally grown and native purple Concorde variety. In the same manner, you are going to get white grape juice, from the indigenous Niagara variety. These are both different from the European varieties. In California, the Sultana variety is normally dried and sold as sun-dried raisins, but sometimes you may also find yourself drinking white juice obtained from the sultanas.

Resveratrol

A grape constituent of red grapes called resveratrol is getting to be very controversial. In the past couple of years, some researchers wanted to find out why people living in the Mediterranean regions, especially in France and in Italy had a lower percentage of heart problems and ailments. They had plenty of fatty food, many of them led sedentary lives, but still they did not bother much about heart attacks, and other such ailments, which should have normally been their lot.

Was it something in their genetic makeup? Well, the answer was found. It was the red grape glass of wine, these men and women took with their meals. The secret magic ingredient is known as Resveratrol. The moment this information got onto the Internet, many enterprising companies began selling products purporting to be original Resveratrol in pill form. There way of giving the general public was that you do not have to eat the original grape, when you can get the same benefit from our [quite expensive] Resveratrol substitute.

Well, if you are spending a lot of money buying something which has been endorsed by a favorite music star, well, it is your loss. Of course, the marketed product is definitely not the original thing, however much the companies may progress that it is. So if you do not get your glass of original rich red wine, made from fresh grapes, grape skin, grape stems and seeds, that means that you are not getting the true Resveratrol.

In the same way, Grape seed oil, and grape seed extract are also being touted about by a number of companies as being excellent for skin care. Well, that is true, but that is because they have linoleic acid, plenty of vitamin E, phytosterols and also oleic acid, which are normally produced chemically by pharmaceutical companies, and sold to other companies making expensive beauty products.

So what is to stop them from adding these products and then marketing it as with original grape seed oil. It has been done.

Christmas Fruitcake

I am really nutty about this particular fruitcake, no pun intended. This is a definite traditional must especially for Christmastime.

For this you need half a cup of preserved and shredded orange peel.
Half a cup of shredded and preserved Citron.
1 cup of candied cherries, cut into half.
Half a pound of light seedless raisins
1 cup of blanched almonds, sly word, and chopped pecans mixed together.
2 teaspoons full of grated lemon rind
2 cups of sifted all-purpose flour
Half a cup of sifted all-purpose flour. Yes, they have been repeated twice, because they are going to be used twice, but in different quantities!
1 teaspoon baking powder
Half a teaspoonful of salt.
1 cup shortening, or butter. You may also use margarine.
1 cup granulated sugar
Five eggs unbeaten
1 teaspoon lemon juice

Shred the orange peel, and the Citron on a vegetable shredder. That is the cherries and poor boiling water over the apricots and raisins. Let them stand for five minutes. Drain them, and then pat them dry between an absorbent towel. Chop the apricots and the pecans.

Grate the lemon rind. Combine with the half cup of flour and mix that well.

Now set the oven at 300°F for preheating. Grease a 10x5x3 cake pan.

Sift together the baking powder, the rest of the flour and the salt.

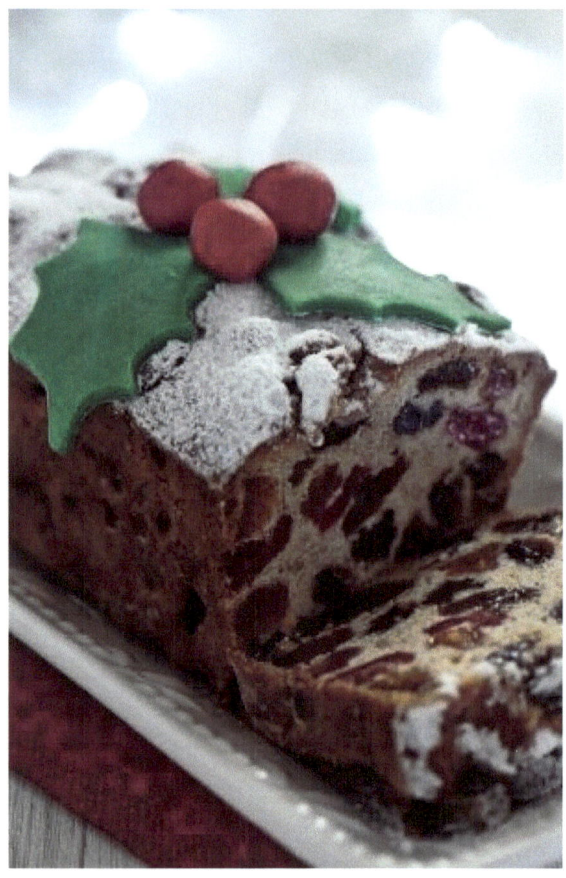

Now add the shortening and the sugar to your blender, and blend for two minutes. Keep adding the eggs one at a time, while beating for another 2 ½ minutes.

Now add the lemon juice and the flour mixture and beat for another one minute, scraping the blender bowl , if necessary, with a wooden scraper.

Then add the fruit and the nut mixture continuously, while beating for about 1 ½ minutes.

Turn this mixture into the pan, and bake for 1hour and 45 minutes. Your cake tester should come out really smoothly.

Cool on a cake rack for half an hour, then remove from the pan. Wrap up and placed in a covered a tight container. You can also refrigerate this.

Traditional Carrot Pudding

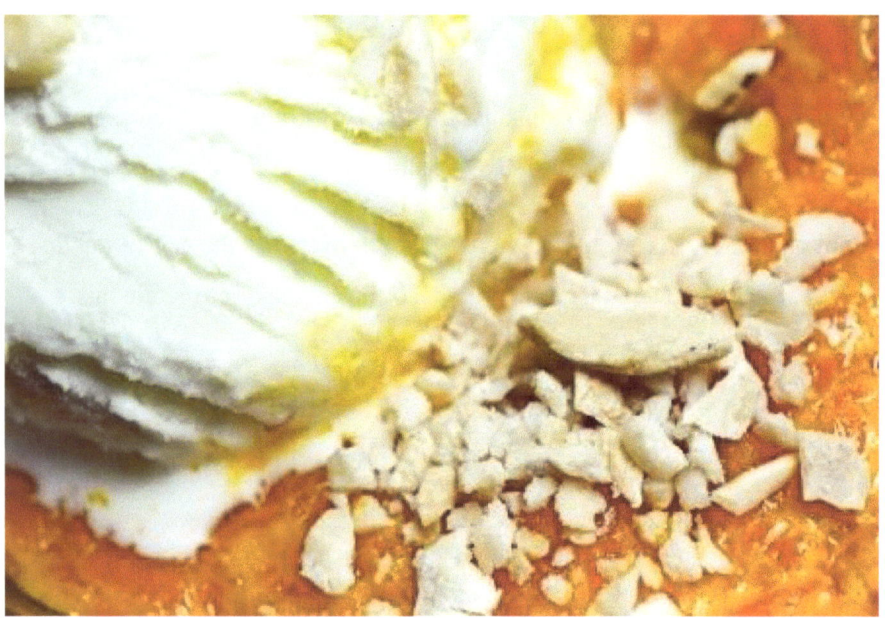

Ingredients –

1 L full cream milk.

1 kg grated carrots.

2 ½ cups of milk.

Four – 5 tablespoons clarified butter, also known as desi ghee. This gives this dish its particular richness, as well as a fragrant luxurious aroma.

Half a cup of sugar

Chopped nuts like raisins, almonds, walnuts, pistachios, as many as you like. The more the merrier.

* Statutory warning – this is not for cholesterol watchers!

Now this is a traditional and very rich Eastern dish, which is normally made up of 1 L of full cream milk, which is poured slowly to boil for half an hour and being stirred continuously. By that time, its volume gets reduced to one third the quantity. Now this is really rich and concentrated milk.

Now, in other saucepan you are going to add 1 kg of grated carrots to 2 ½ cups of milk and cook for 20 minutes, until the milk nearly dries out. Add the sugar, and mix well. Cook in the remaining liquid, until this pudding turns dry.

Add the clarified butter. Now, mix well, and add the concentrated milk. Mix well again, and stir on a low heat, until you feel the wok turning greasy on its sides. That is because of the clarified butter being separated from the main cooked carrots.

Once that is done, it means your dish is ready to serve. Mix the chopped nuts and remove from the fire. Sprinkle more raisins and the rest of the nuts on top of this pudding, before serving hot.

Well, I happen to like lots of cream and lots of butter, like Julia Child. So I normally add one tablespoonful of fresh cream over the pudding, and well, I am in foodie heaven.

Using Grapes for Natural Cures

Constipation

Suffering from constipation? Add grape juice to your diet. Small children suffering from constipation can get relief, if you give them one teaspoonful of grape juice. This is going to get their system moving.

Teething Problems

 In the same manner, if they are suffering from teething pains, just keep feeding them a spoonful of grape juice, along with a mixture of half a teaspoonful of ground roasted cumin seeds boiled in water.

Stress and Strain

Now this is a good remedy for all those people were suffering from tension, stress and strain. Just make sure that a few raisins are added to a glassful of hot milk and boiled. Then drink it down with a teaspoonful of honey added. This is normally a winter recipe, so drink it only in the winter.

TB

People suffering from tuberculosis have shown a marked improvement, when they were given plenty of red grape juice in large quantities.

Dry Cough

A dry cough can be cured by taking 10 g each of powdered almonds, licorice, and raisins. Grind them together, and make small pellets with a little bit of honey. Now take two of the pellets at a time and suck them to get rid of that dry cough. Make sure that the raisins are unseeded.

Flatulence and Digestion Related Problems

If you are suffering from digestion related problems, all you have to do is take 50 g fresh juice of grapes, first thing in the morning. You are soon going to find your digestion working perfectly. One tablespoonful of liquid is about 16 g. So you need 3 tablespoons and a little bit over. Follow up with a fistful of grapes.

Conclusion

So now that you know all about grapes, and their varieties, as well as their historical importance down the ages, enjoy your grapes, and stay healthy!

Live long and prosper!

Author Bio

Dueep Jyot Singh is a Management and IT Professional who managed to gather Postgraduate qualifications in Management and English and Degrees in Science, French and Education while pursuing different enjoyable career options like being an hospital administrator, IT,SEO and HRD Database Manager/ trainer, movie scriptwriter, theatre artiste and public speaker, lecturer in French, Marketing and Advertising, ex-Editor of Hearts On Fire (now known as Solstice) Books Missouri USA, advice columnist and cartoonist, publisher and Aviation School trainer, ex- moderator on Medico.in, banker, student councilor ,travelogue writer … among other things!

One fine morning, she decided that she had enough of killing herself by Degrees and went back to her first love -- writing. It's more enjoyable! She already has 48 published academic and 14 fiction- in- different- genre books under her belt.

When she is not designing websites or making Graphic design illustrations for clients , she is browsing through old bookshops hunting for treasures, of which she has an enviable collection – including R.L. Stevenson, O.Henry, Dornford Yates, Maurice Walsh, C.N.Williamson, Sapper, Bartimeus and the crown of her collection- Dickens "The Old Curiosity Shop," and so on… Just call her "Renaissance Woman" - collecting herbal remedies, acting like Universal Helping Hand/Agony Aunt, or escaping to her dear mountains for a bit of exploring, collecting herbs and plants, and trekking.

Check out some of the other JD-Biz Publishing books

Health Learning Series

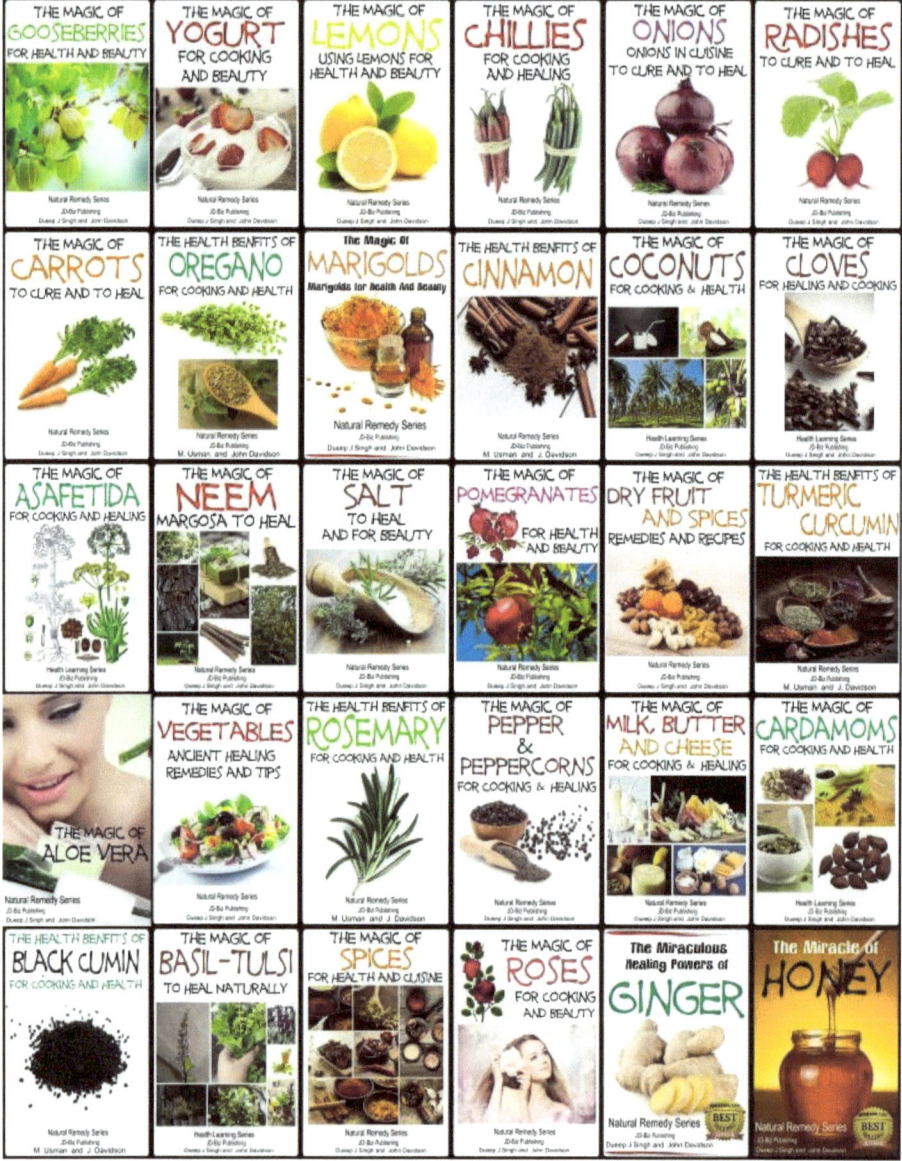

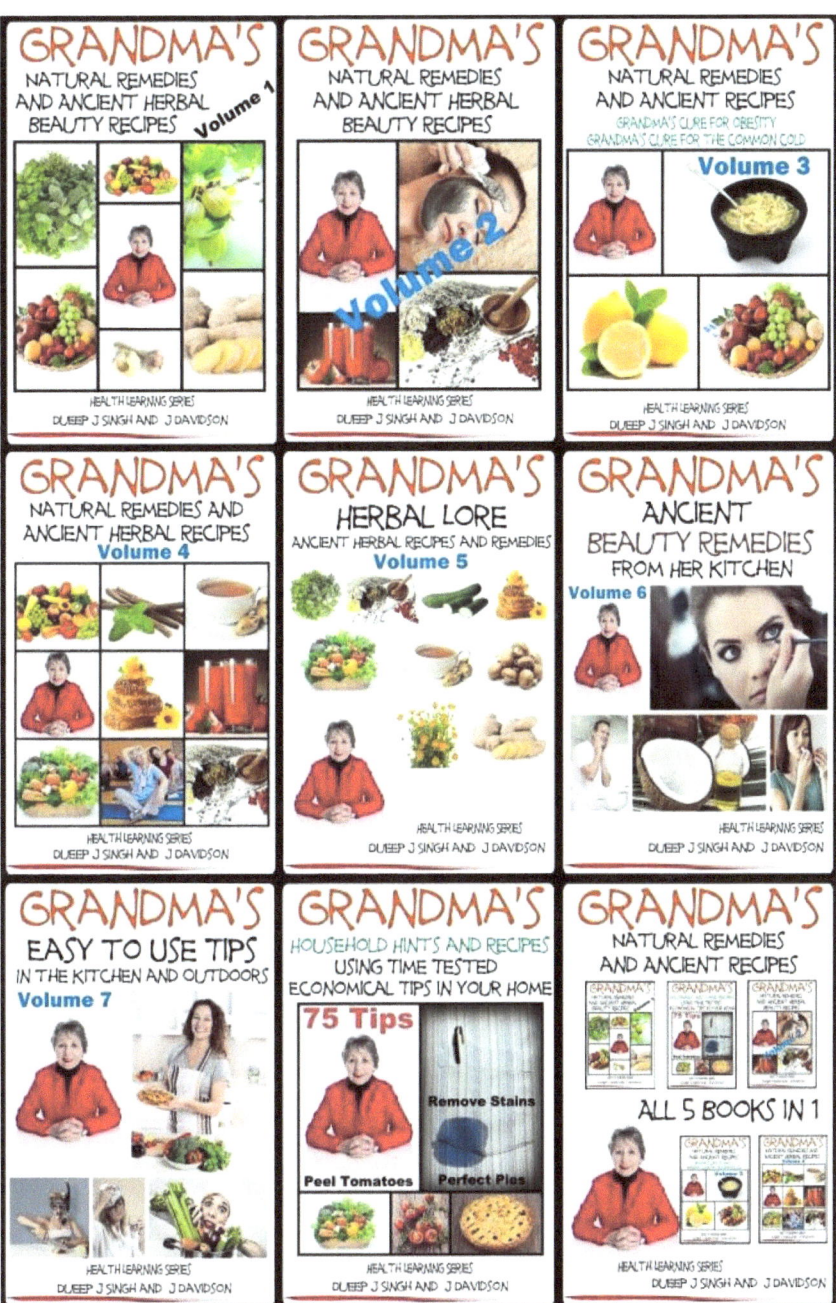

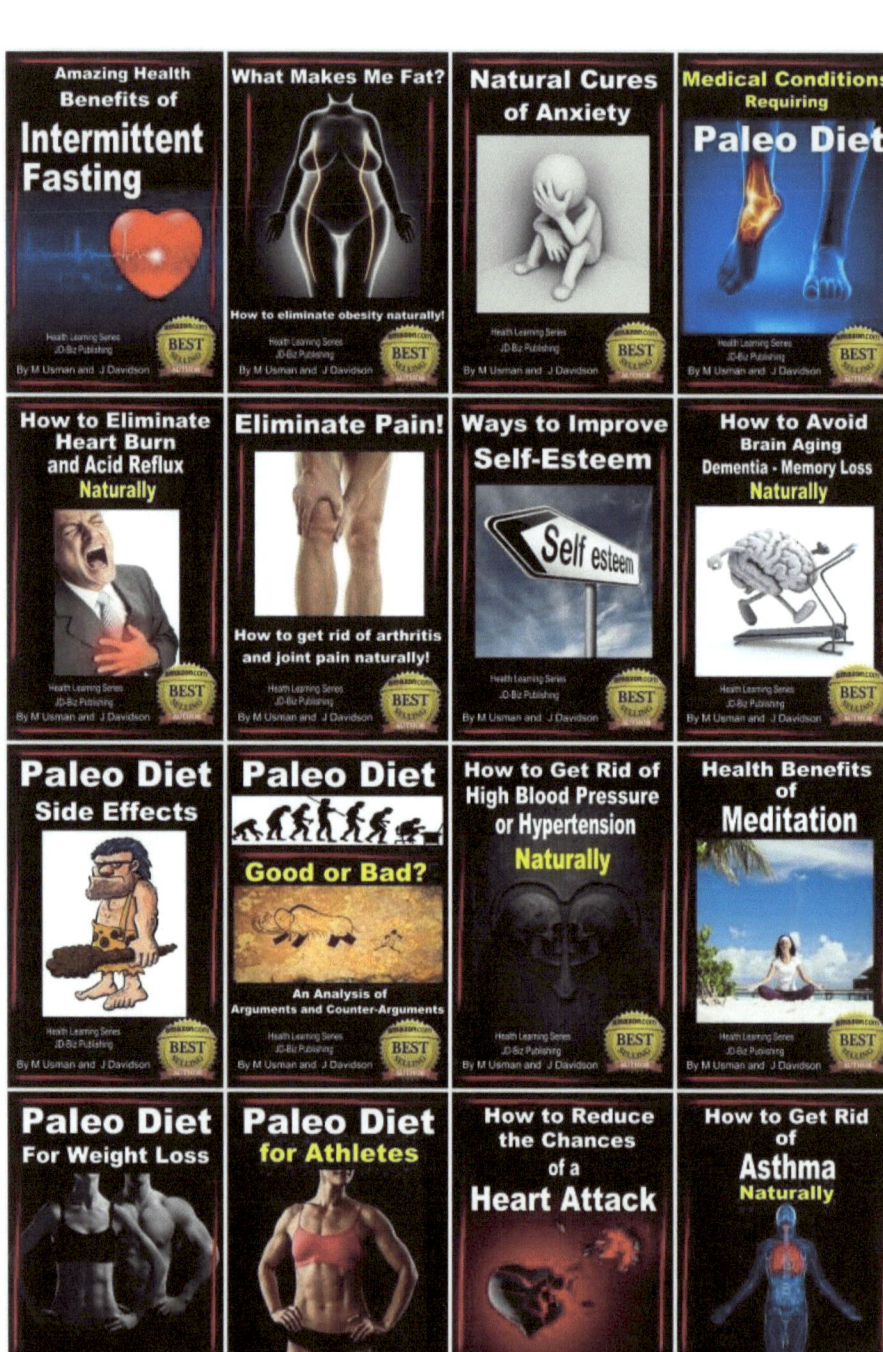

Amazing Animal Book Series

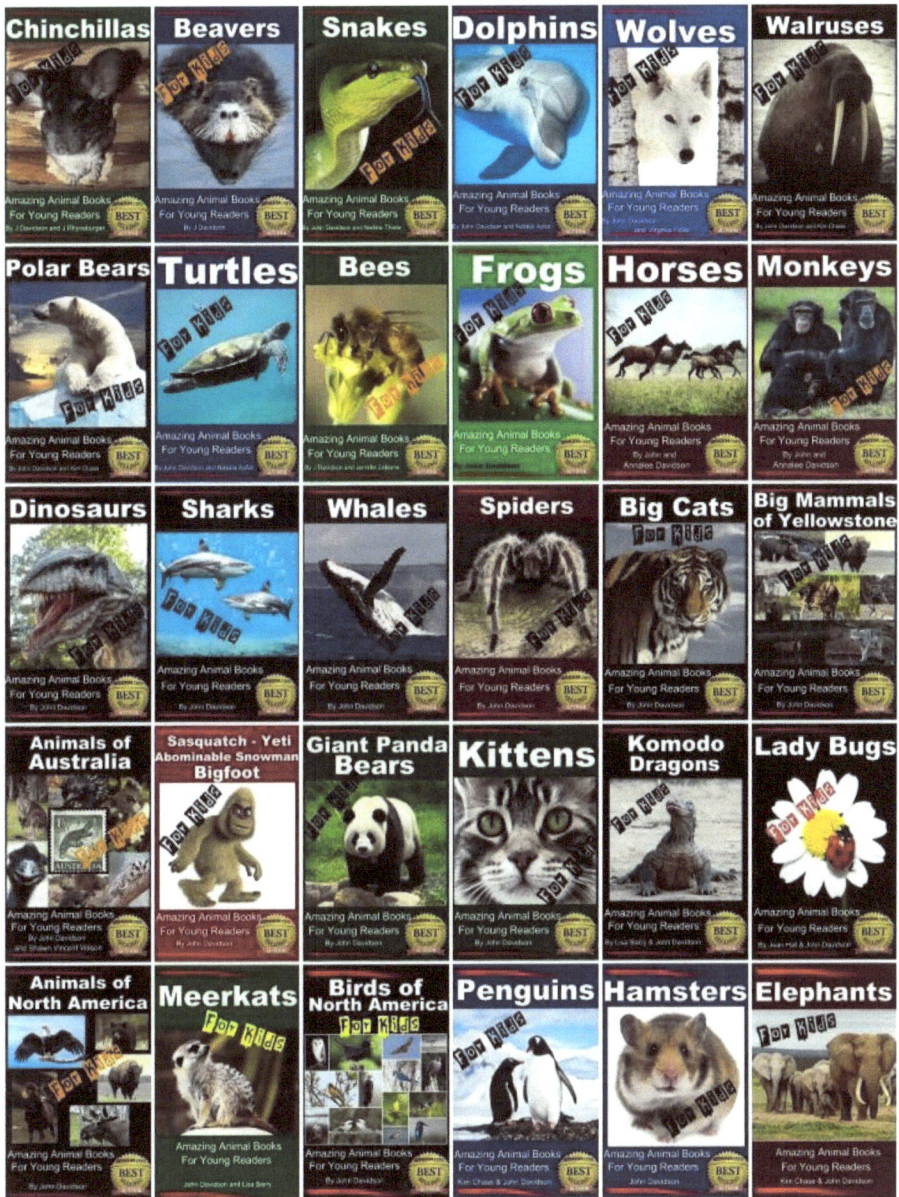

Learn To Draw Series

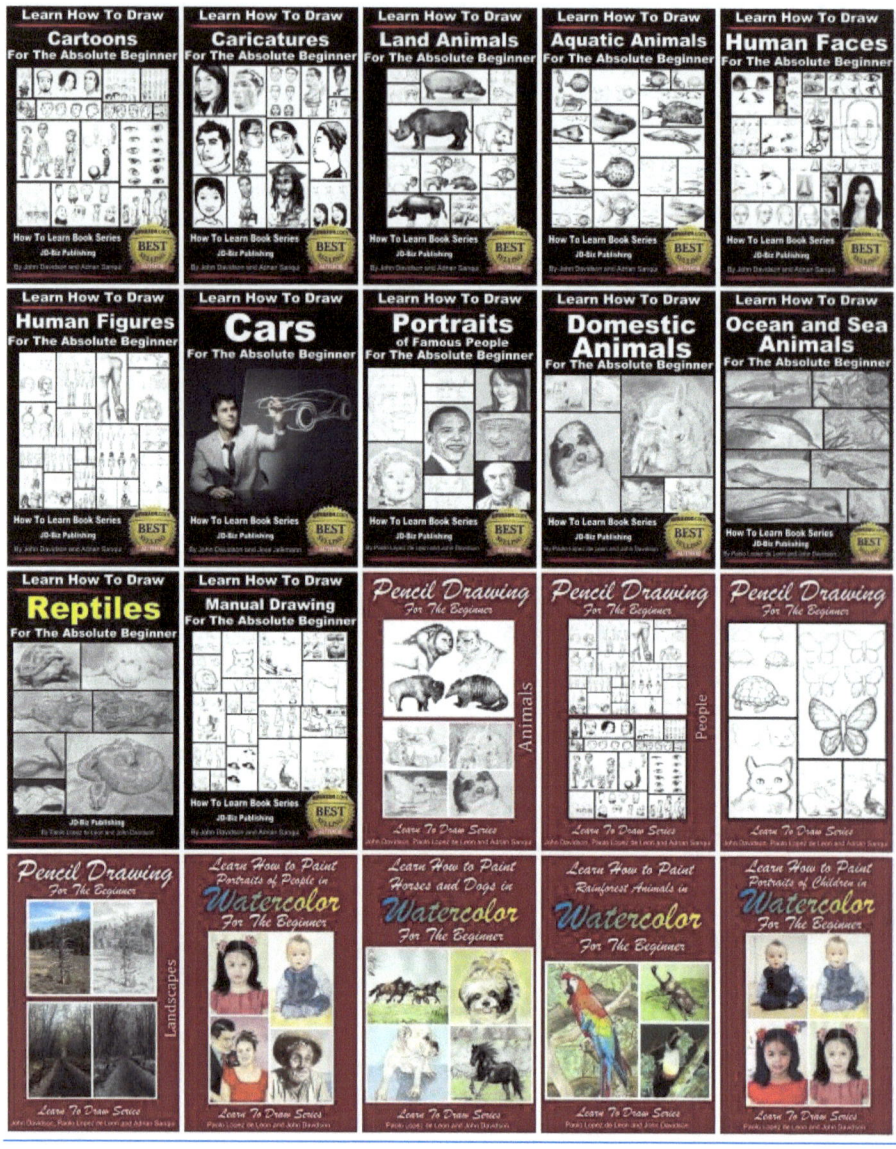

How to Build and Plan Books

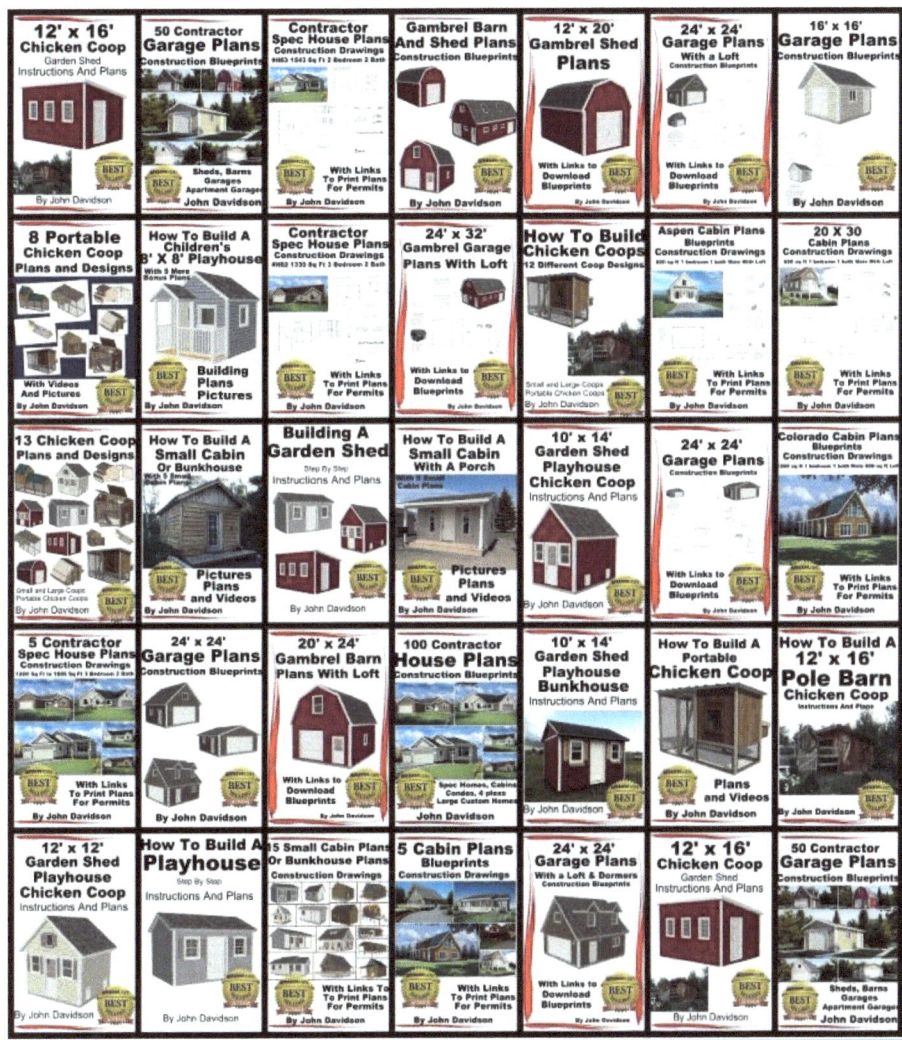

Entrepreneur Book Series

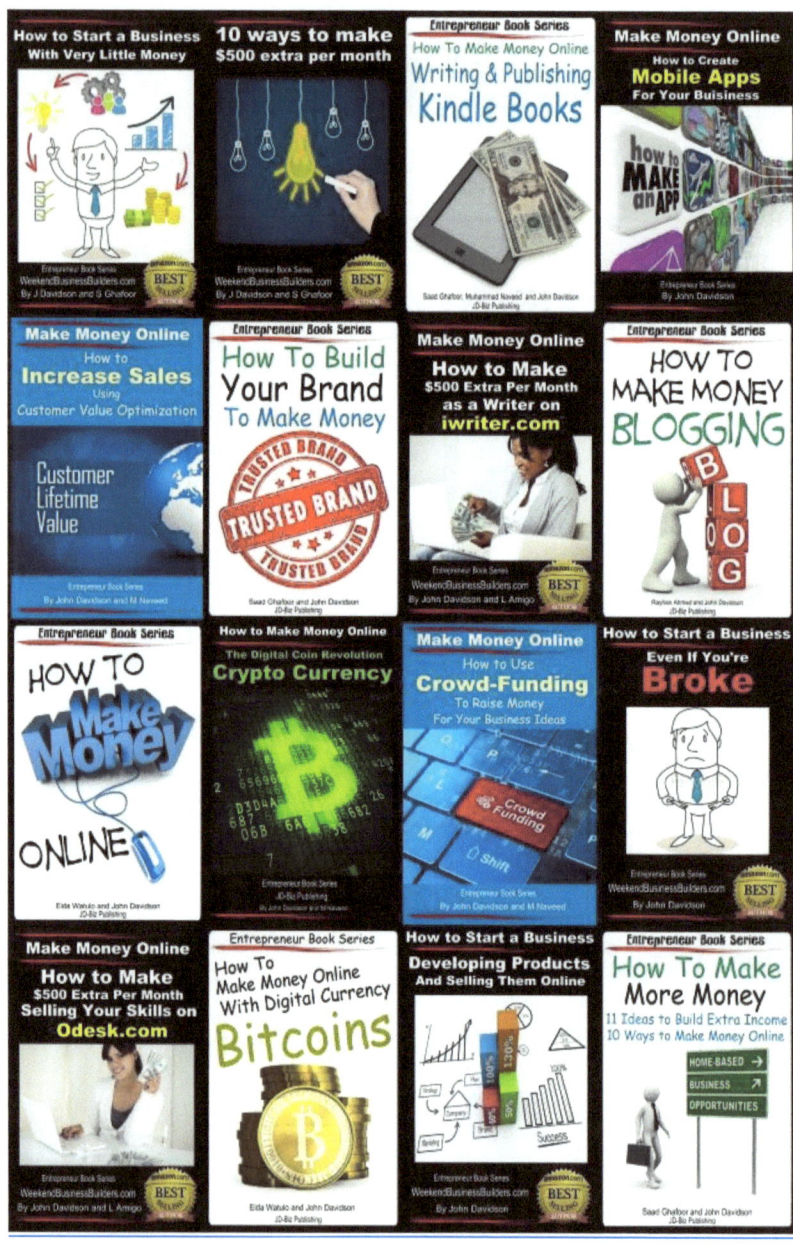

Our books are available at

1. Amazon.com

2. Barnes and Noble

3. Itunes

4. Kobo

5. Smashwords

6. Google Play Books

Download Free Books!

http://MendonCottageBooks.com

Publisher

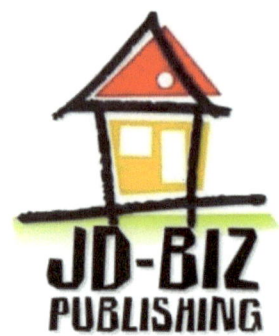

JD-Biz Corp

P O Box 374

Mendon, Utah 84325

http://www.jd-biz.com/

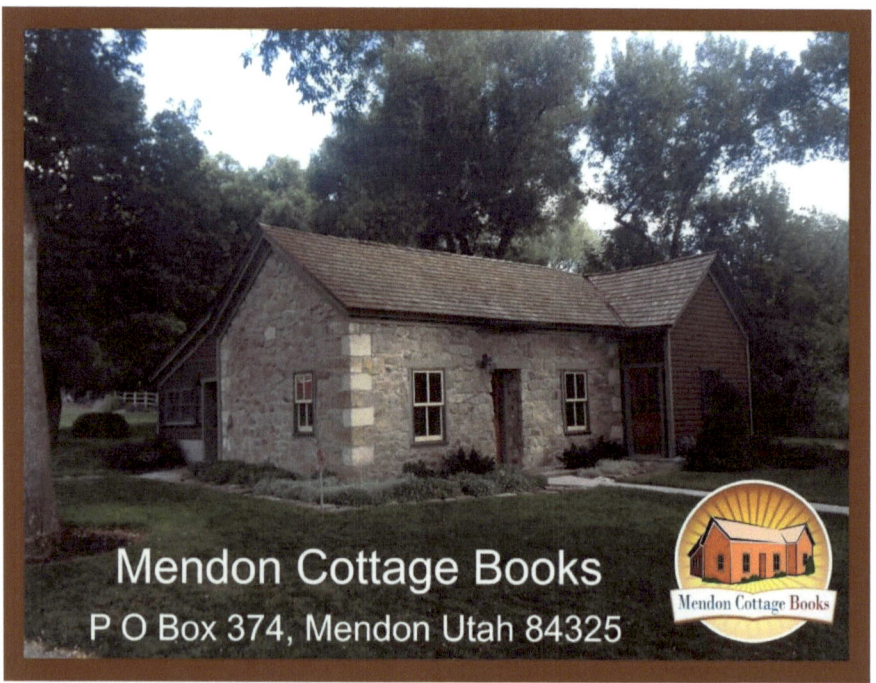

Mendon Cottage Books

P O Box 374, Mendon Utah 84325

www.ingramcontent.com/pod-product-compliance
Lightning Source LLC
Chambersburg PA
CBHW050836290526
45792CB00001B/416